EASY STRETCHING EXERCISE FOR SENIORS OVER 60

Discover the key to staying active and independent in your golden years with these senior-friendly stretching exercises."

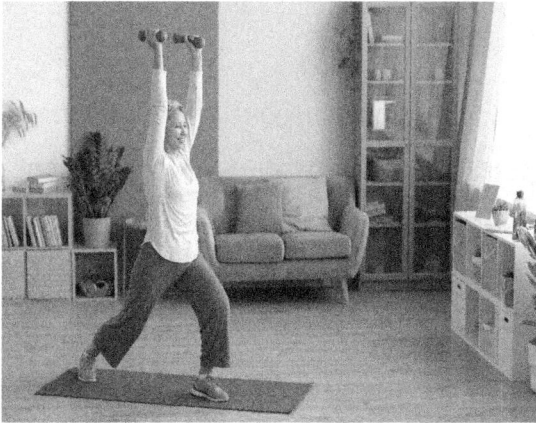

Raul G. Lake

Copyright © 2024 Raul G. lake

This publication contains easy stretching exercises tailored for seniors over 60, designed to promote flexibility, mobility, and overall well-being. While every effort has been made to ensure the accuracy and effectiveness of the exercises, readers are advised to consult with a healthcare professional before beginning any exercise program, especially if they have any pre-existing health conditions or concerns

TABLE OF CONTENTS

INTRODUCTION

As we age, it becomes increasingly important to pay attention to our physical health and well-being. One key component of maintaining a healthy and active lifestyle as a senior is incorporating regular stretching exercises into our daily routine. Stretching not only helps improve flexibility, but it can also reduce the risk of injury, alleviate muscle tension, and improve overall mobility.

In this guide, we will explore easy stretching exercises specifically designed for seniors over the age of 60. Whether you are new to stretching or have been practicing it for some time, this guide will provide you with a variety of stretches targeting different parts of the body and offer tips on how to safely and effectively incorporate them into your daily routine.

By committing to a regular stretching routine, you can improve your quality of life, maintain independence, and feel better both physically and mentally. So, let's get started on this journey to a healthier and more active lifestyle through stretching exercises for seniors.

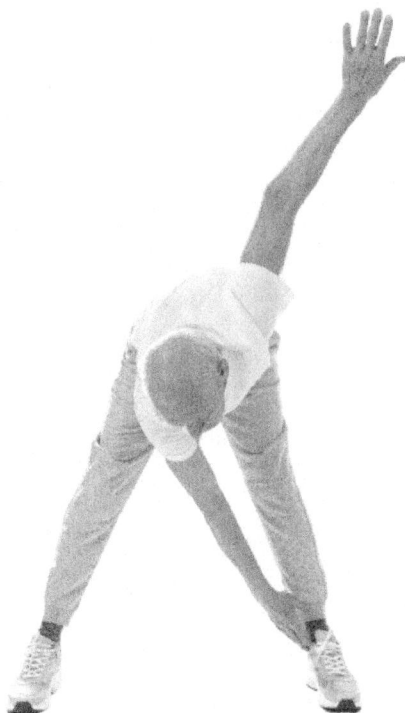

ONE

IMPORTANCE OF STRETCHING FOR SENIORS

As we age, our bodies undergo various changes, including a decrease in muscle mass, flexibility, and joint mobility. These age-related changes can make everyday activities more challenging and increase the risk of injury. This is where the importance of stretching for seniors comes into play.

Stretching exercises are vital for seniors for several reasons:

1. Improved Flexibility: Regular stretching helps to increase flexibility in the muscles and joints, making it easier to perform daily tasks such as bending, reaching, and turning without straining or injuring the muscles.

2. Enhanced Range of Motion: Stretching exercises can help seniors maintain or improve their range of motion, allowing them to move more freely and with less discomfort. This can be especially beneficial for seniors with conditions such as arthritis or joint stiffness.

3. Injury Prevention: Stretching before and after physical activity can help seniors reduce the risk of muscle strains, sprains, and other injuries by warming up the muscles and improving blood circulation to the tissues.

4. Improved Posture: Stretching exercises can help seniors maintain good posture by reducing muscle tension and stiffness in the back, shoulders, and neck. Good posture can prevent back pain and improve overall body alignment.

5. Stress Relief: Stretching can also have mental health benefits for seniors, helping to reduce stress, improve mood, and promote relaxation. This mind-body connection can contribute to overall well-being and quality of life.

6. Better Balance and Coordination: Stretching exercises that focus on stability and balance can help seniors improve their balance and coordination, reducing the risk of falls and enhancing mobility.

Incorporating stretching exercises into a daily routine can have significant benefits for seniors, enhancing their physical health, preventing injuries, and promoting overall well-being. It is essential for seniors to consult with their healthcare provider or a fitness professional before starting any new exercise routine to ensure that the stretches are safe and appropriate for their individual needs and health conditions. Stretching is a simple yet effective way for seniors to maintain independence, improve mobility, and enjoy an active and healthy lifestyle.

Benefits of Stretching for Seniors

Stretching exercises offer a multitude of benefits for seniors, making them an essential component of a healthy and active lifestyle. Here are some key benefits of stretching for seniors:

1. Improved Flexibility: Stretching helps to lengthen and loosen tight muscles, improving flexibility and range of motion. Better flexibility makes it easier to perform daily activities such as bending down, reaching for objects, and getting in and out of chairs or beds.

2. Enhanced Muscle Function: Regular stretching can help seniors maintain and improve muscle function, strength, and endurance. Strong and flexible muscles are essential for mobility and independence as we age.

3. Pain Relief: Stretching exercises can alleviate muscle tension, reduce stiffness, and decrease joint pain in seniors. Stretching can help to relieve discomfort from conditions such as arthritis, back pain, and sciatica.

4. Improved Posture and Balance: Stretching helps to lengthen and relax muscles, promoting good posture and spinal alignment. Better posture can reduce the risk of falls and improve balance and stability in seniors.

5. Stress Reduction: Engaging in stretching exercises can have a calming effect on the mind and body, reducing stress and promoting relaxation. This can help seniors feel more at ease, improve mood, and enhance overall well-being.

6. Better Circulation: Stretching increases blood flow to the muscles, improving circulation and oxygen delivery to the tissues. Improved circulation can help prevent muscle cramps, reduce swelling, and promote healing in seniors.

7. Injury Prevention: Regular stretching can help seniors prevent injuries by improving muscle flexibility and joint mobility. Stretching before and after physical activity can warm up the muscles and reduce the risk of strains, sprains, and other injuries.

8. Enhanced Quality of Life: Incorporating stretching exercises into a daily routine can enhance the quality of life for seniors by promoting physical health, mental well-being, and independence. Stretching can help seniors stay active, mobile, and engaged in their daily activities.

In conclusion, stretching exercises offer numerous benefits for seniors, including improved flexibility, muscle function, pain relief, posture, balance, stress reduction, circulation, injury prevention, and overall quality of life. Seniors can enjoy these benefits by incorporating stretching into their daily routine, staying active, and maintaining a healthy and active lifestyle. Always consult with a healthcare provider or fitness professional before beginning any new exercise program to ensure that the stretches are safe and appropriate for individual needs and health conditions.

Common Age-Related Issues That Stretching Can Help Improve

As we age, our bodies undergo various changes that can impact our physical health and mobility. Stretching exercises are a valuable tool for seniors to combat age-related issues and maintain a healthy and active lifestyle. Here are some common age-related issues that stretching can help improve:

1. Decreased Flexibility: Aging can lead to a gradual decrease in flexibility, which can result in stiffness in the muscles and joints. Regular stretching helps to improve flexibility by lengthening the muscles and increasing range of motion, making it easier to move and perform daily activities.

2. Joint Stiffness: Seniors often experience joint stiffness due to changes in cartilage and connective tissues. Stretching exercises can help to reduce joint stiffness by increasing blood flow to the joints, lubricating them, and improving overall joint health.

3. Muscle Weakness: Loss of muscle mass and strength is a common age-related issue that can affect balance, mobility, and independence. Stretching helps to maintain and improve muscle strength by increasing blood flow to the muscles, promoting muscle growth, and enhancing muscle function.

4. Poor Posture: Aging can contribute to poor posture, characterized by a rounded back, forward head posture, and hunched shoulders. Stretching exercises targeting the muscles of the back, neck, and shoulders can help to improve posture, reduce muscle tension, and promote spinal alignment.

5. Reduced Balance and Stability: Seniors may experience a decline in balance and stability, increasing the risk of falls and injuries. Stretching exercises that focus on balance, coordination, and stability can help seniors improve their balance, reduce the risk of falls, and enhance mobility.

6. Back Pain: Chronic back pain is a common age-related issue that can affect seniors' quality of life. Stretching exercises that target the muscles of the back, hips, and core can help to alleviate back pain, reduce muscle tension, and improve spinal alignment.

7. Arthritis: Arthritis is a common condition among seniors that causes joint pain, stiffness, and inflammation. Stretching exercises can help alleviate arthritis symptoms by increasing joint flexibility, improving circulation, and reducing pain and stiffness in the affected joints.

8. Circulation Issues: Aging can lead to reduced circulation, which can result in muscle cramps, swelling, and slow healing of injuries. Stretching exercises that promote blood flow to the muscles can help improve circulation, prevent muscle cramps, reduce swelling, and promote healing in seniors.

Incorporating stretching exercises into a regular routine can help seniors address common age-related issues, improve flexibility, muscle strength, posture, balance, and overall quality of life. It is essential for seniors to consult with a healthcare provider or fitness professional before starting any new exercise program to ensure that the stretches are safe and suitable for individual needs and health conditions. Stretching is a simple yet effective way for seniors to maintain mobility, independence, and well-being as they age.

Tips for Safe and Effective Stretching

Stretching is a beneficial and essential component of a senior's fitness routine, helping to improve flexibility, mobility, and overall well-being. To ensure a safe and effective stretching experience, consider the following tips:

1. Warm Up: Before starting your stretching routine, warm up your muscles with gentle physical activity such as walking or marching in place. This helps to increase blood flow to the muscles and prepare them for stretching.

2. Start Slow: Begin your stretching session with gentle and gradual movements, focusing on slow and controlled stretches. Avoid bouncing or jerking movements, as this can lead to muscle strain or injury.

3. Listen to Your Body: Pay attention to how your body feels during stretching. Stretch to a point of mild tension, not pain. If you experience sharp or intense pain, stop the stretch immediately and consult with a healthcare provider.

4. Hold Each Stretch: Hold each stretch for 15-30 seconds, breathing deeply and slowly throughout the stretch. Avoid holding your breath and try to relax the muscles being stretched.

5. Focus on Major Muscle Groups: Target major muscle groups in your stretching routine, including the hamstrings, quadriceps, calves, hips, shoulders, and back. Include both static stretches (holding a position) and dynamic stretches (moving through a range of motion).

6. Stretch Both Sides: Make sure to stretch both sides of the body evenly to maintain balance and symmetry. If one side feels tighter than the other, spend extra time stretching that side to improve flexibility.

7. Stay Consistent: Consistency is key to seeing the benefits of stretching. Aim to stretch at least 2-3 times per week to maintain and improve flexibility and mobility.

8. Use Props and Modifications: Consider using props such as a chair, wall, or strap to assist with stretching exercises, especially if you have limited flexibility or mobility. Modify stretches as needed to accommodate any physical limitations or health conditions.

9. Cool Down: After completing your stretching routine, cool down with gentle movements and deep breathing to help relax the muscles and reduce muscle soreness.

10. Consult with a Professional: If you're new to stretching or have specific health concerns, consider consulting with a fitness professional or physical therapist for personalized guidance and recommendations.

By following these tips for safe and effective stretching, seniors can enjoy the benefits of improved flexibility, reduced muscle tension, and enhanced mobility while minimizing the risk of injury. Remember that consistency, proper technique, and listening to your body are key factors in a successful stretching routine. Enjoy the benefits of stretching and stay active as you age!

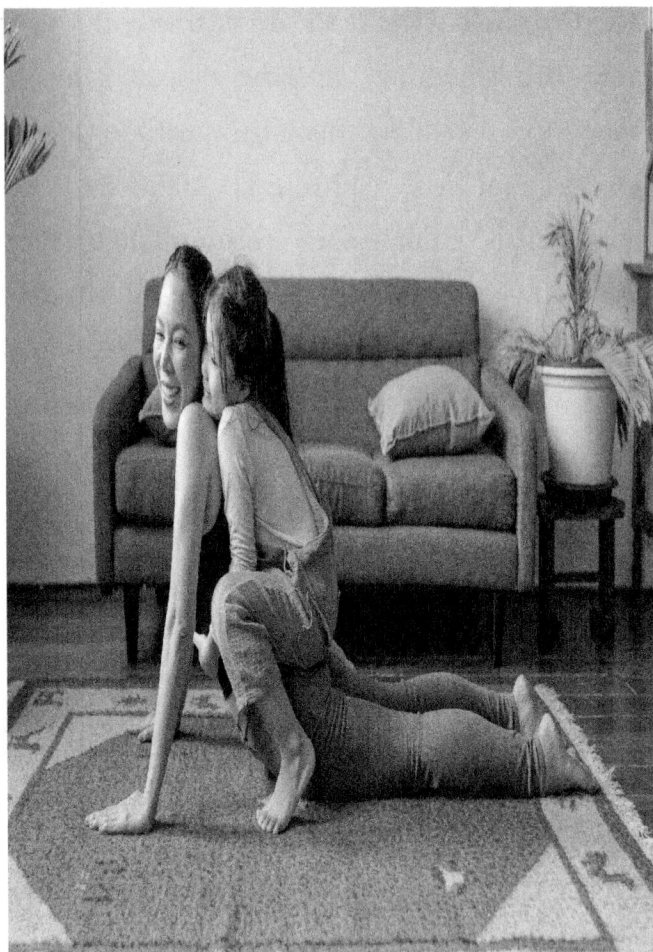

TWO:

GETTING STARTED WITH STRETCHING

Starting a stretching routine as a senior can be a beneficial and rewarding experience, promoting flexibility, mobility, and overall well-being. Here are some helpful tips to get you started with stretching:

1. Consult with Your Healthcare Provider: Before starting any new exercise routine, including stretching, it's essential to consult with your healthcare provider or a fitness professional. They can provide guidance on exercises that are safe and appropriate for your individual needs and health conditions.

2. Set Realistic Goals: Determine your goals for stretching, whether it's improving flexibility, reducing muscle tension, or enhancing mobility. Set realistic and achievable goals to help keep you motivated and track your progress.

3. Create a Safe Space: Find a comfortable and safe space to perform your stretching routine. Make sure the area is well-lit, free of obstacles, and provides enough room to move and stretch freely.

4. Wear Comfortable Clothing: Wear loose, comfortable clothing that allows for easy movement during stretching exercises. Avoid wearing tight or restrictive clothing that may limit your range of motion.

5. Use Proper Equipment: Depending on your flexibility and mobility, you may need to use props or equipment such as a yoga mat, chair, strap, or foam roller to assist with stretching exercises. These tools can help you achieve proper alignment and deepen your stretches safely.

6. Start Slow: Begin your stretching routine with gentle and simple stretches targeting major muscle groups. Focus on areas that feel tight or tense, and gradually increase the intensity and duration of your stretches over time.

7. Incorporate Breathing: Remember to breathe deeply and slowly during each stretch, inhaling as you lengthen the muscles and exhaling as you release tension. Deep breathing can help promote relaxation and enhance the benefits of stretching.

8. Be Mindful of Your Body: Pay attention to how your body feels during stretching. If you experience pain, discomfort, or dizziness, stop the stretch immediately and listen to your body's signals. Modify the stretch or seek guidance from a healthcare provider if needed.

9. Stay Hydrated: Drink water before and after your stretching routine to stay hydrated and help maintain muscle function and flexibility.

10. Be Consistent: Aim to incorporate stretching into your daily routine, whether it's in the morning, before physical activity, or as part of your bedtime routine. Consistency is key to seeing improvements in flexibility and mobility over time.

By following these tips and guidelines, seniors can safely and effectively start a stretching routine to improve flexibility, reduce muscle tension, and enhance overall well-being. Remember to listen to your body, set realistic goals, and enjoy the benefits of stretching as you progress on your fitness journey.

Preparing for a Stretching Routine

Before embarking on a stretching routine as a senior, it's important to take some preparatory steps to ensure a safe and effective experience. These are some tips that can help you to prepare for a stretching routine:

1. Warm Up: Before starting your stretching routine, it's essential to warm up your muscles with light aerobic exercises such as walking, marching in place, or gentle cycling. This helps increase blood flow to the muscles and prepares them for stretching.

2. Choose a Comfortable Environment: Select a quiet and spacious area in your home or a well-ventilated room where you can stretch comfortably. Make sure the space is free of clutter and provides enough room to move and stretch without any obstacles.

3. Wear Suitable Attire: Dress in agreeable, baggy apparel that considers unlimited development during extending works out. Abstain from wearing tight or constrictive dress that might restrict your scope of movement.

4. Gather Equipment: Depending on your flexibility and mobility level, you may need props or equipment such as a yoga mat, chair, strap, or foam roller to assist with certain stretching exercises. Have these items nearby to support you during your routine.

5. Hydrate: Drink water before and after your stretching routine to stay hydrated and maintain muscle function. Proper hydration is essential for overall health and well-being, including during exercise.

6. Check Your Posture: Before starting each stretch, ensure proper posture by standing or sitting tall with your spine aligned. Good posture helps maximize the effectiveness of your stretches and reduces the risk of injury.

7. Set Realistic Goals: Determine your goals for stretching, whether it's improving flexibility, reducing muscle tension, or enhancing mobility. Establish realistic and achievable goals to keep you motivated and track your progress.

8. Make a Daily schedule: Foster an organized extending schedule that incorporates an assortment of stretches focusing on various muscle gatherings. Center around unique stretches to heat up the muscles and static stretches to increment adaptability and protract muscles.

9. Listen to Your Body: Throughout your stretching routine, pay attention to how your body feels. If you experience pain, discomfort, or strain, adjust the stretch or stop and seek guidance from a healthcare provider.

10. Breathe and Relax: Remember to breathe deeply and calmly during each stretch, inhaling as you lengthen the muscles and exhaling as you relax into the stretch. Deep breathing helps promote relaxation and enhance the benefits of stretching.

By following these preparation tips, seniors can ensure a safe and effective stretching routine that promotes flexibility, mobility, and overall well-being. With proper warm-up, equipment, hydration, posture, and goal-setting, you can set the stage for a rewarding and enjoyable stretching experience. Enjoy the process and reap the benefits of improved flexibility and mobility as you incorporate stretching into your daily routine.

Finding a Comfortable and Safe Space to Stretch

Making an agreeable and place of refuge for extending is fundamental for seniors hoping to further develop adaptability, versatility, and in general prosperity. Here are a few hints to assist you with tracking down the ideal region to extend easily and securely:

1. Choose a Quiet Environment: Select a quiet and peaceful environment where you can focus on your stretching routine without distractions or interruptions. Choose a spot away from noisy areas or high traffic areas to create a relaxing space for stretching.

2. Ensure Ample Space: Find a room or area with enough room to move freely and perform stretching exercises without feeling restricted. Clear the space of any furniture or obstacles that may impede your movements during stretching.

3. Optimal Lighting: Make sure the space is well-lit to prevent tripping or straining your eyes during stretching exercises. Natural light or bright overhead lighting can help create a welcoming and inviting atmosphere for stretching.

4. Comfortable Flooring: look for a comfortable and safe place to stretch on, such as a yoga mat, carpet, or padded floor. A cushioned surface can help cushion your joints and provide support during floor-based stretches.

5. Proper Ventilation: Ensure the room is well-ventilated with fresh air to keep you comfortable and prevent overheating during your stretching routine. Open windows or use a fan to improve air circulation and maintain a comfortable temperature.

6. Access to Props: Have any necessary props or equipment nearby, such as a chair, yoga block, strap, or foam roller, to assist with certain stretches or provide added support during your stretching routine.

7. Peaceful Atmosphere: Create a peaceful and soothing atmosphere in your stretching space by playing calming music, lighting scented candles, or practicing mindfulness techniques to promote relaxation and focus.

8. Maintain Safety: Prioritize safety during stretching by choosing a space free of tripping hazards, sharp objects, or loose items that could cause accidents. Make sure the area is clear and safe for movement and stretching.

9. Personalization: Personalize your stretching space to suit your preferences and needs. Add personal touches such as inspiring quotes, plants, or decorative elements that create a positive and motivating environment for your stretching routine.

10. Enjoy the Experience: Make the most of your stretching space by infusing it with positivity, comfort, and relaxation. Take time to unwind, breathe deeply, and appreciate the benefits of stretching in a comfortable and safe environment.

By following these tips, seniors can make an agreeable and place of refuge for extending that upgrades the experience and advances a positive and pleasant daily practice. Whether it's in a committed room, a calm corner of your home, or a tranquil open air setting, finding the right space for extending can have a massive effect on your adaptability, portability, and by and large prosperity. Partake all the while and embrace the advantages of extending in an agreeable and safe climate customized to your necessities and inclinations.

How often and how long to stretch

Stretching is an important component of a senior's fitness routine, promoting flexibility, mobility, and overall well-being. To maximize the achievement of stretching, it's crucial to understand how often to stretch and how long to hold each stretch. Here are some guidelines to help you develop a safe and effective stretching routine:

Frequency of Stretching:

- Aim to stretch at least 2-3 times per week to maintain and improve flexibility. Consistency is key to seeing progress and reaping the benefits of stretching.

- Consider incorporating stretching into your daily routine, such as in the morning, before physical activity, or as part of your bedtime routine. Regular stretching can help prevent muscle stiffness and improve range of motion.

Duration of Stretching:

- Hold each stretch for 15-30 seconds to allow the muscles to lengthen and relax. Avoid bouncing or jerking movements, as this can lead to muscle strain.

- Focus on a slow and controlled stretch, feeling a gentle pull or tension in the muscle. If you experience discomfort or pain, ease off the stretch immediately.

- Repeat each stretch 2-3 times on each side to maximize flexibility and range of motion. Gradually increase the duration of your stretches as your flexibility improves.

Dynamic vs. Static Stretching:

- Dynamic stretching involves moving through a range of motion to warm up the muscles and improve flexibility before physical activity. Perform dynamic stretches before exercise to prepare the body for movement.

- Static stretching involves holding a position for a set period to elongate and relax the muscles. Incorporate static stretches into your routine to improve flexibility, reduce muscle tension, and enhance mobility.

Listen to Your Body:- Pay attention to how your body responds to stretching and adjust the intensity or duration of stretches accordingly. Stretch to a point of mild tension, not pain, and breathe deeply and slowly throughout each stretch.

- If you experience sharp or intense pain, stop the stretch immediately and consult with a healthcare provider. Modify stretches as needed to accommodate any physical limitations or health conditions.

By following these guidelines for how often and how long to stretch, seniors can develop a safe and effective stretching routine that promotes flexibility, mobility, and overall well-being. Remember to stay consistent, listen to your body, and enjoy the benefits of stretching as you progress on your fitness journey. Incorporate stretching into your routine regularly to maintain and improve flexibility, enhance mobility, and support a healthy and active lifestyle.

THREE:

upper body stretch

Stretching the upper body is essential for seniors to improve
adaptability, diminish muscle strain, and improve by and large portability. Incorporating upper body stretches into your routine can help alleviate stiffness and promote better posture. Here are some effective upper body stretches for seniors:

1. Shoulder Stretch:

- Stand or sit tall with your shoulders loose

- Reach one arm across your body and use the other arm to gently press it closer to your chest.

- Hold the stretch for 15-30 seconds, feeling a gentle stretch in the shoulder and upper back.

- Switch arms and repeat on the other side.

2. Neck Stretch:

- Sit or stand with a tall posture.

- Gently tilt your head to one side, bringing your ear towards your shoulder.

- Hold the stretch for 15-30 seconds, feeling a stretch along the side of your neck.

- Repeat on the other side, then gently tilt your head forward and backward to stretch different neck muscles.

3. Triceps Stretch:

- Raise one arm above your head and bend your elbow, reaching your hand down towards your upper back.

- Use your other hand to gently press the elbow for a deeper stretch in the triceps.

- Hold the stretch for 15-30 seconds, feeling the stretch along the back of your arm.

- Switch arms and repeat on the other side.

4. Chest Stretch:

- Stand tall with your shoulders relaxed.

- Clasp your hands behind your back and straighten your arms.

- Lift your arms slightly and open your chest, feeling a stretch in the chest and shoulders.

- Hold the stretch for 15-30 seconds, then release.

5. Upper Back Stretch:

- Sit on a chair or stand with your feet hip-width apart.

- Clasp your hands in front of you and round your back, pushing your hands away and dropping your head.

- Hold the stretch for 15-30 seconds, feeling a stretch in the upper back and shoulders.

- Release and repeat as needed.

6. Arm Circles:

- Stand with your arms out to the sides at shoulder height.

- Begin making circular motions with your arms, gradually increasing the size of the circles.

- Reverse the direction of the circles after a few repetitions.

- Continue for 30 seconds to warm up the shoulders and arms.

Remember to breathe deeply and focus on relaxing into each stretch. Hold each stretch for 15-30 seconds and repeat on both sides to balance the upper body. Incorporate these upper body stretches into your daily routine to improve flexibility, reduce muscle tension, and enhance mobility as a senior. Consult with a healthcare provider or fitness professional before starting any new exercise routine, especially if you have any underlying health conditions or concerns. Enjoy the benefits of stretching and maintain a healthy and active lifestyle through regular upper body stretches.

NECK STRETCHES

Title: The Ultimate Guide to Neck Stretches: Relieving Tension and Enhancing Mobility

1. Neck Tilt:

- Sit or stand comfortably with your spine erect and shoulders relaxed.

- Slowly tilt your head towards one shoulder, aiming to bring your ear closer to your shoulder without straining.

- Hold the stretch for 15-30 seconds, feeling the gentle stretch along the opposite side of your neck.

- Return to the starting position and repeat on the other side.

- Perform 2-3 sets on each side, breathing deeply throughout the stretch.

2. Neck Rotation:

- Begin in a neutral position with your head facing forward.

- Slowly rotate your head to one side, trying to bring your chin over your shoulder.

- Hold the stretch for 15-30 seconds, feeling the tension release in the neck muscles.

- Return to the center and repeat on the other side.

- Complete 2-3 sets on each side, maintaining smooth and controlled movements.

3. Neck Flexion and Extension:

- Sit or stand tall, keeping your shoulders relaxed.

- Gently lower your chin towards your chest, feeling a stretch along the back of your neck.

- Hold this position for 15-30 seconds, focusing on elongating the spine.

- Slowly lift your head upward, tilting it back slightly to stretch the front of your neck.

- Hold for another 15-30 seconds, being mindful of any discomfort.

- Repeat the sequence 2-3 times, moving with awareness and breathing deeply.

4. Shoulder Shrugs:

- Relax your arms by your sides and take a deep breath in.

- Lift your shoulders towards your ears as you inhale, creating tension in the neck and shoulder muscles.

- Hold for a moment, then exhale as you gently release the tension and lower your shoulders down.

- Repeat this motion 8-10 times, allowing the breath to guide the movement.

- Focus on letting go of any tension with each exhale, promoting relaxation in the neck and shoulders.

5. Side Neck Stretch:

- Sit or stand tall, maintaining good posture.

- Reach one arm down towards the ground and place the opposite hand on the top of your head.

- Slowly tilt your head to the side, guiding your ear towards your shoulder until you feel a stretch along the side of your neck.

- Hold the stretch for 15-30 seconds, breathing deeply into the stretch.

- Switch sides and repeat, aiming for 2-3 sets on each side to balance the stretch.

Shoulder stretches

Shoulder extends are significant for seniors to further develop adaptability, diminish firmness, and improve scope of movement in the shoulders and chest area. Integrating shoulder extends into your routine can assist with forestalling shoulder agony and distress, particularly for seniors who might encounter snugness in the shoulders because of maturing or dormancy. Here are some viable shoulder extends for seniors:

1. Shoulder Roll:

- Sit or remain with your shoulders free.

- Gradually roll your shoulders forward in a roundabout movement, lifting them up towards your ears, then, at that point, back and down.

- Rehash the shoulder rolls for 10-15 times, then, at that point, turn around the course and roll your shoulders in reverse.

2. Shoulder Stretch Across the Chest:

- Stand or sit tall with your shoulders free.

- Arrive at your right arm across your chest, utilizing your passes available to press the right arm nearer to your body delicately.

- Hold the stretch for 15-30 seconds, feeling a stretch in the shoulder and upper back.

- Rehash on the opposite side by bringing your left arm across your chest and utilizing your right hand to help with the stretch.

3. Shoulder Stretch with a Lash:

- Hold a lash, towel, or belt with two hands behind your back.

- Open your chest and fix your arms, lifting the lash marginally to extend the shoulders.

- save the stretch for fifteen to thirty seconds, feeling a delicate stretch toward the front of the shoulders and chest.

- Delivery and rehash on a case by case basis.

4. Arm Circles:

- Stand with your arms out to the sides at shoulder level.

- Start making roundabout movements with your arms, continuously expanding the size of the circles.

- Invert the heading of the circles after a couple of reiterations.

- Go on for 30 seconds to heat up the shoulders and further develop versatility.

5. Above Shoulder Stretch:

- Sit or stand tall with your shoulders free.

- Arrive at the two arms above and fasten your hands together.

- Tenderly lift your arms up towards the roof, feeling a stretch in the shoulders and upper back.

- Hold the stretch for 15-30 seconds, then deliver and rehash on a case by case basis.

6. Shoulder Bone Press:

- Sit or remain with your shoulders free.

- Press your shoulder bones together as though attempting to hold a pencil between them.

- Hold the crush for 5-10 seconds, then, at that point, discharge.

- Rehash the shoulder bone crush for 10-15 reiterations to reinforce the upper back and further develop the act.

Make sure to inhale profoundly, loosen up your muscles, and move delicately through each stretch. Hold each stretch for 15-30 seconds and rehash on the two sides to adjust the shoulders. Integrate these shoulder extends into your day to day daily practice to further develop adaptability, diminish shoulder strain, and upgrade versatility as a senior. Talk with a medical care supplier or wellness proficient prior to beginning any new work-out daily practice, particularly on the off chance that you have any basic ailments or concerns. Partake in the advantages of shoulder extends and keep up with sound shoulders and chest area versatility through normal extending works out

Arm And Wrist Stretches For Seniors

Arm and wrist extends are significant for seniors to further develop adaptability, lessen pressure, and forestall distress in the furthest points. Integrating arm and wrist extends into your everyday schedule can assist with keeping up with portability and capability in the arms, hands, and wrists, particularly for seniors who might encounter solidness or agony because of joint pain or dreary developments. Here are some successful arm and wrist extends for seniors:

1. Wrist Flexor Stretch:

- Broaden your right arm forward with the palm confronting.

- Utilize your passed close by to push down on the fingers of the right hand, feeling a stretch along the highest point of the wrist and lower arm delicately.

- Hold the stretch for 15-30 seconds, then switch sides and rehash on the left arm.

2. Wrist Extensor Stretch:

- Broaden your right arm forward with the palm looking up.

- Utilize your passed close by to push down on the rear of the hand, feeling a stretch along the underside of the wrist and lower arm tenderly.

- Hold the stretch for 15-30 seconds, then switch sides and rehash on the left arm.

3. Lower arm Stretch:

- Broaden your right arm forward with the palm overcoming.

- Utilize your pass close by to tenderly twist the wrist vertically, feeling a stretch in the lower arm and wrist.

- Hold the stretch for 15-30 seconds, then switch sides and rehash on the left arm.

4. Rear arm muscle Stretch:

- Arrive at your right arm above and curve the elbow, bringing the give over towards the back.

- Utilize your passed close by to delicately push on the elbow, feeling a stretch in the rear arm muscle.

- Hold the stretch for 15-30 seconds, then, at that point, switch sides and rehash on the left arm.

5. Bicep Stretch:

- Stretch out your right arm out to the side with the palm looking up.

- Utilize your passed close by to tenderly press the fingers of the right give over and internal, feeling a stretch in the bicep muscle.

- Hold the stretch for 15-30 seconds, then, at that point, switch sides and rehash on the left arm.

6. Arm Circles:

- Stand with your arms out to the sides at shoulder level.

- Start making round movements with your arms, slowly expanding the size of the circles.

- Invert the course of the circles after a couple of redundancies.

- Go on for 30 seconds to heat up the arms and shoulders.

Make sure to move delicately and easily through each stretch, breathing profoundly and zeroing in on unwinding. Hold each stretch for 15-30 seconds and rehash on the two sides to keep up with balance in the arms and wrists. Integrate these arm and wrist extends into your day to day everyday practice to further develop adaptability, lessen muscle pressure, and improve versatility as a senior. Talk with a medical services supplier or wellness proficient prior to beginning any new work-out everyday practice, particularly on the off chance that you have any basic medical issue or concerns. Partake in the advantages of arm and wrist extends and keep up with solid and portable furthest points through normal extending works out

Chest And Upper Back Stretches Are

Significant for seniors to further develop act, decrease snugness, and advance adaptability in the chest area. Integrating chest and upper back extends into your routine can assist with reducing strain, further develop scope of movement, and forestall uneasiness in the shoulders and back. Here are some compelling stretches for seniors to focus on the chest and upper back:

1. Chest Opener Stretch:

- Stand tall with your feet hip-width separated.

- Fasten your hands behind your back and fix your arms.

- Lift your arms marginally and open your chest, feeling a stretch in the chest and shoulders.

- Hold the stretch for 15-30 seconds, then, at that point, discharge.

2. Upper Back Stretch:

- Sit on a seat or stand with your feet hip-width separated.

- Fasten your hands before you and round your back, driving your hands away and dropping your head.

- Hold the stretch for 15-30 seconds, feeling a stretch in the upper back and shoulders.

- Delivery and rehash depending on the situation.

3. Situated Shoulder Bone Press:

- Sit tall in a seat with your shoulders loose.

- Crush your shoulder bones together as though attempting to hold a pencil between them.

- Hold the press for 5-10 seconds, then, at that point, discharge.

- Rehash the shoulder bone press for 10-15 redundancies to reinforce the upper back and further develop pose.

4. Feline Cow Stretch:

- Start on all fours in a tabletop position.

- Breathe in as you curve your back, dropping your stomach towards the floor and lifting your head and tailbone towards the roof (Cow present).

- Breathe out as you round your back, tucking your jaw to your chest and squeezing your hands into the floor (Feline posture).

- Stream among Feline and Cow models for a couple of breaths to extend the chest, upper back, and spine.

5. Entryway Chest Stretch:

- Stand in an entryway with your arms at shoulder level and elbows bowed at 90 degrees.

- Step forward with one foot to make a delicate stretch in the chest and shoulders.

- Hold the stretch for 15-30 seconds, then switch sides and rehash.

6. Side Stretch:

- Sit or stand tall with your arms broadened above.

- Arrive at one arm over-top to the contrary side, feeling a stretch at the edge of the body.

- Hold the stretch for 15-30 seconds, then switch sides and rehash.

Make sure to move gradually and carefully through each stretch, breathing profoundly and zeroing in on unwinding. Hold each stretch for 15-30 seconds and rehash on the two sides to equitably focus on the chest and upper back. Consolidate these stretches into your day to day daily practice to further develop, diminish pressure, and improve portability in the chest area as a senior. Talk with a medical services supplier or wellness proficient prior to beginning any new work-out daily schedule, particularly in the event that you have any basic medical issue or concerns. Partake in the advantages of chest and upper back extends and keep major areas of strength for a portable chest area through standard extending works out.

FOUR:

LOWER BODY STRETCHES

Stretching the lower body is essential for seniors to improve flexibility, reduce muscle tension, and enhance mobility in the hips, legs, and lower back. Incorporating lower body stretches into your routine can help alleviate stiffness, improve balance, and reduce the risk of falls. Here are some effective stretches for seniors to target the lower body:

1. Hamstring Stretch:

- Sit on the edge of a chair with one leg extended straight out in front of you.

- Flex your foot and hinge at the hips to lean forward slightly, feeling a stretch in the back of the extended leg.

- Hold the stretch for 15-30 seconds, then switch legs and repeat.

2. Quadriceps Stretch:

- Stand tall with one hand on a chair or wall for support.

- Bend one knee and grasp your ankle with your hand, bringing your heel towards your glutes.

- Keep your knees close together and gently push your hip forward to deepen the stretch in the front of the thigh.

- Hold the stretch for 15-30 seconds, then switch legs and repeat.

3. Hip Flexor Stretch:

- Kneel on a cushioned surface with one foot forward and the knee bent at a 90-degree angle.

- Engage your core and shift your weight forward, feeling a stretch in the front of the hip and thigh.

- Hold the stretch for 15-30 seconds, then switch legs and repeat.

4. Calf Stretch:

- Stand facing a wall with your hands resting on the wall for support.

- Step one foot back and press the heel into the floor, keeping the back leg straight and the front knee bent.

- Lean forward into the stretch, feeling a stretch in the calf muscle of the back leg.

- Hold the stretch for 15-30 seconds, then switch legs and repeat.

5. Inner Thigh Stretch:

- Sit on the floor with your back straight and legs extended out to the sides in a straddle position.

- Lean forward from the hips, keeping your back straight and chest lifted, feeling a stretch in the inner thighs and groin.

- Hold the stretch for 15-30 seconds, then sit back up.

6. Glute Stretch:

- Lie on your back and bend both knees, placing one ankle over the opposite knee.

- Reach through the space between your legs and clasp your hands behind the thigh of the bottom leg.

- Gently pull the knee towards your chest, feeling a stretch in the hip and glutes.

- Hold the stretch for 15-30 seconds, then switch legs and repeat.

Remember to breathe deeply and relax into each stretch, focusing on maintaining proper alignment and avoiding any pain. Hold each stretch for 15-30 seconds and repeat on both sides to target the lower body evenly. Incorporate these lower body stretches into your daily routine to improve flexibility, reduce muscle tension, and enhance mobility as a senior. Consult with a healthcare provider or fitness professional before starting any new exercise routine, especially if you have any underlying health conditions or concerns. Enjoy the benefits of lower body stretches and maintain a strong and mobile lower body through regular stretching exercises.

Hip Stretches For Seniors

Hip stretches are crucial for seniors to improve flexibility, reduce tightness, and maintain mobility in the hip joints. The hips play a significant role in everyday movements such as walking, sitting, and standing, making it important to keep them flexible and healthy. Incorporating hip stretches into your routine can help prevent hip pain, improve hip function, and reduce the risk of injuries. Here are some effective hip stretches for seniors:

1. Hip Flexor Stretch:

- Kneel on one knee with the opposite foot flat on the floor in front of you.

- Engage your core and shift your weight forward, feeling a stretch in the front of the hip and thigh.

- Hold the stretch for 15-30 seconds, then switch legs and repeat.

2. Pigeon Pose:

- Start in a tabletop position on your hands and knees.

- Bring your right knee forward towards your right wrist and extend your left leg straight back behind you.

- Lower your hips towards the floor, feeling a deep stretch in the outer hip and glutes.

- Hold the stretch for 15-30 seconds, then switch sides and repeat.

3. Figure Four Stretch:

- Sit on the edge of a chair with your feet flat on the floor.

- Cross your right ankle over your left knee, creating a "figure four" shape with your legs.

- Lean forward slightly, feeling a stretch in the hip and glutes of the crossed leg.

- Hold the stretch for 15-30 seconds, then switch legs and repeat.

4. Seated Hip Stretch:

- Sit on the floor with your legs extended out in front of you.

- Bend one knee and cross it over the opposite leg, placing the foot flat on the floor.

- Twist your torso towards the bent knee, using your opposite elbow to gently press against the knee, feeling a stretch in the hip and lower back.

- Hold the stretch for 15-30 seconds, then switch sides and repeat.

5. IT Band Stretch:

- Stand with your feet hip-width apart and cross your right leg behind the left.

- Reach your right arm overhead and lean towards the left, feeling a stretch along the outer hip and thigh.

- Hold the stretch for 15-30 seconds, then switch sides and repeat.

6. Hip Circles:

- Stand tall with your hands on your hips.

- Circle your hips in a clockwise direction, focusing on fluid and controlled movements.

- Reverse the direction and circle your hips in a counterclockwise motion.

- Continue for 30 seconds to loosen up the hip joints and improve mobility.

Remember to move mindfully and gently through each stretch, breathing deeply and focusing on relaxation. Hold each stretch for 15-30 seconds and repeat on both sides to target the hips evenly. Incorporate these hip stretches into your daily routine to improve hip flexibility, reduce tightness, and maintain healthy hip function as a senior. Consult with a healthcare provider or fitness professional before starting any new exercise routine, especially if you have any underlying health conditions or concerns. Enjoy the benefits of hip stretches and keep your hips mobile and pain-free through regular stretching exercises.

Leg and Calf Stretches for Seniors

Leg and calf stretches are essential for seniors to improve flexibility, reduce muscle tension, and maintain range of motion in the lower body. Incorporating leg and calf stretches into your daily routine can help prevent stiffness, improve circulation, and reduce the risk of injuries in the legs and calves. Here are some effective stretches for seniors to target the legs and calves:

1. Standing Quad Stretch:

- Stand tall with your feet hip-width apart.

- Bend your right knee and grasp your right ankle with your right hand, bringing your heel towards your glutes.

- Keep your knees close together and gently push your hip forward, feeling a stretch in the front of the thigh.

- Hold the stretch for 15-30 seconds, then switch legs and repeat.

2. Standing Calf Stretch:

- Stand facing a wall with your hands resting on the wall for support.

- Step one foot back and press the heel into the floor, keeping the back leg straight and the front knee bent.

- Lean forward into the stretch, feeling a stretch in the calf muscle of the back leg.

- Hold the stretch for 15-30 seconds, then switch legs and repeat.

3. Seated Leg Extension Stretch:

- Sit on the floor with your legs extended out in front of you.

- Reach for your toes or ankles, keeping your back straight and chest lifted, feeling a stretch in the back of the legs (hamstrings).

- Hold the stretch for 15-30 seconds, then sit back up.

4. Standing Hamstring Stretch:

- Stand with your feet hip-width apart.

- Hinge at the hips and bend forward, reaching towards your toes or shins.

- Keep your back straight and avoid rounding the spine, feeling a stretch in the back of the legs (hamstrings).

- Hold the stretch for 15-30 seconds, then slowly come back up.

5. Calf Stretch with Wall:

- Stand facing a wall and place your hands on the wall at shoulder height.

- Step one foot back and press the heel into the floor, keeping the back leg straight.

- Lean forward into the wall, feeling a stretch in the calf muscle of the back leg.

- Hold the stretch for 15-30 seconds, then switch legs and repeat.

6. Leg and Ankle Circles:

- Sit on a chair with your feet flat on the floor.

- Lift one leg and make circular motions with your foot and ankle in a clockwise direction.

- Reverse the direction and make circles in a counterclockwise motion.

- Continue for 30 seconds, then switch legs and repeat.

Remember to breathe deeply and relax into each stretch, focusing on maintaining proper alignment and avoiding any pain. Hold each stretch for 15-30 seconds and repeat on both sides to target the legs and calves evenly. Incorporate these leg and calf stretches into your daily routine to improve flexibility, reduce muscle tension, and maintain healthy lower body function as a senior. Consult with a healthcare provider or fitness professional before starting any new exercise routine, especially if you have any underlying health conditions or concerns. Enjoy the benefits of leg and calf stretches and keep your lower body strong and mobile through regular stretching exercises.

Ankle and Foot Stretches for Seniors

Ankle and foot stretches are important for seniors to improve flexibility, reduce the risk of falls, and maintain mobility in the lower extremities. The ankles and feet play a crucial role in balance, stability, and overall lower body function, making it essential to keep them strong and flexible. Incorporating ankle and foot stretches into your routine can help prevent stiffness, improve range of motion, and alleviate discomfort in the ankles and feet. Here are some effective stretches for seniors to target the ankles and feet:

1. Calf Stretch with Towel:

- Sit on the floor with your legs extended out in front of you.

- Loop a towel around the ball of one foot and gently pull the towel towards you, feeling a stretch in the calf muscle.

- Hold the stretch for 15-30 seconds, then switch feet and repeat.

2. Plantar Fascia Stretch:

- Sit on a chair and place one foot over your opposite knee.

- Hold the base of your toes and gently pull them back towards you, feeling a stretch on the bottom of the foot (plantar fascia).

- Hold the stretch for 15-30 seconds, then switch feet and repeat.

3. Ankle Circles:

- Sit on a chair with your feet flat on the floor.

- Lift one foot off the ground and rotate your ankle in a circular motion, first clockwise and then counterclockwise.

- Continue for 30 seconds, then switch feet and repeat.

4. Toe Flexion and Extension:

- Sit on a chair with your feet flat on the floor.

- Curl your toes towards the sole of your foot, holding for a few seconds, then extend your toes upwards, feeling a stretch in the toes and the top of the foot.

- Repeat the flexion and extension movement for 10-15 repetitions on each foot.

5. Heel Cord Stretch:

- Face a wall and place your hands on the wall for support.

- Step one foot back, keeping the heel on the ground and the knee straight.

- Lean forward, feeling a stretch in the calf muscle and Achilles tendon.

- Hold the stretch for 15-30 seconds, then switch feet and repeat.

6. Toe Stretch:

- Sit on a chair with one foot crossed over the opposite knee.

- Interlace your fingers between your toes and gently spread them apart, feeling a stretch in the toes and the bottom of the foot.

- Hold the stretch for 15-30 seconds, then switch feet and repeat.

Remember to move slowly and mindfully through each stretch, breathing deeply and focusing on relaxation. Hold each stretch for 15-30 seconds and repeat on both sides to target the ankles and feet evenly. Incorporate these ankle and foot stretches into your daily routine to improve flexibility, reduce stiffness, and maintain healthy ankle and foot function as a senior. Consult with a healthcare provider or fitness professional before starting any new exercise routine, especially if you have any underlying health conditions or concerns. Enjoy the benefits of ankle and foot stretches and keep your lower extremities strong and mobile through regular stretching exercises.

Full Body Stretches for Seniors

Full body stretches are essential for seniors to improve flexibility, reduce muscle tension, and enhance overall mobility and range of motion. Incorporating full body stretches into your daily routine can help increase blood flow, improve posture, and reduce the risk of injury. Stretching the entire body can also help alleviate stiffness, improve balance, and enhance quality of life. Here are some effective full body stretches for seniors to target all major muscle groups:

1. Neck Stretch:

- Sit or stand tall with your shoulders relaxed.

- Tilt your head to one side, bringing your ear towards your shoulder, feeling a stretch in the side of your neck.

- Hold the stretch for 15-30 seconds, then switch sides and repeat.

2. Shoulder Stretch:

- Extend one arm across your body at shoulder height.

- Use your other hand to gently press the arm towards you, feeling a stretch in the shoulder and upper back.

- Hold the stretch for 15-30 seconds, then switch arms and repeat.

3. Spinal Twist:

- Sit on a chair with your feet planted on the floor.

- Twist your torso to one side, placing one hand on the opposite knee and the other hand on the back of the chair, feeling a stretch in the spine and lower back.

- Hold the stretch for 15-30 seconds, then twist to the other side and repeat.

4. Chest Opener:

- Stand tall with your feet hip-width apart.

- Clasp your hands behind your back and straighten your arms, lifting them slightly and opening up the chest.

- Hold the stretch for 15-30 seconds, feeling a stretch in the chest and shoulders.

5. Seated Forward Fold:

- Sit on the floor with your legs extended out in front of you.

- Hinge at the hips and fold forward, reaching for your toes or shins, feeling a stretch in the back of the legs (hamstrings).

- Hold the stretch for 15-30 seconds, then slowly sit back up.

6. Hip Flexor Stretch:

- Kneel on one knee with the opposite foot flat on the floor in front of you.

- Engage your core and shift your weight forward, feeling a stretch in the front of the hip and thigh.

- Hold the stretch for 15-30 seconds, then switch legs and repeat.

7. Calf Stretch:

- Stand facing a wall with your hands resting on the wall for support.

- Step one foot back and press the heel into the floor, keeping the back leg straight and the front knee bent.

- Lean forward into the stretch, feeling a stretch in the calf muscle of the back leg.

- Hold the stretch for 15-30 seconds, then switch legs and repeat.

8. Seated Spinal Stretch:

- Sit on the floor with your legs crossed.

- Reach your left arm across your body and twist to the right, placing your right hand on the floor behind you, feeling a stretch in the spine and obliques.

- Hold the stretch for 15-30 seconds, then twist to the other side and repeat.

Remember to breathe deeply and relax into each stretch, focusing on proper alignment and avoiding any pain. Hold each stretch for 15-30 seconds and repeat on both sides to target all major muscle groups in the body. Incorporate these full body stretches into your daily routine to improve flexibility, reduce muscle tension, and enhance overall mobility and function as a senior. Consult with a healthcare provider or fitness professional before starting any new exercise routine, especially if you have any underlying health conditions or concerns. Enjoy the benefits of full body stretches and keep your entire body strong, flexible, and mobile through regular stretching exercises

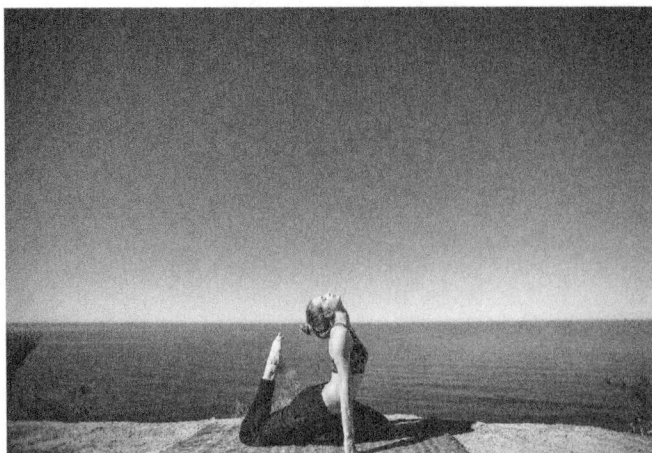

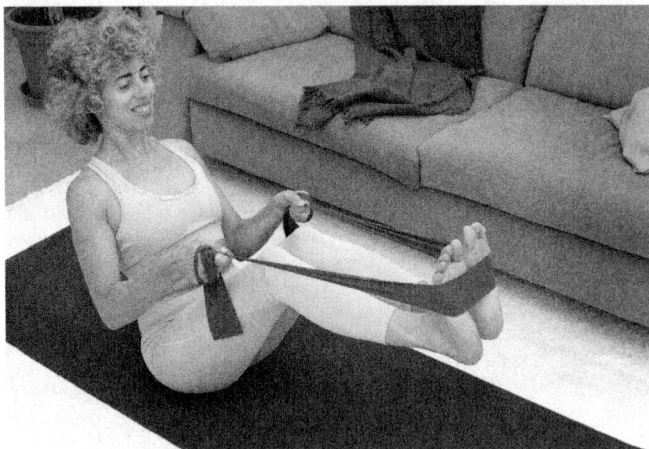

FIVE :

FULL BODY STRETCHES

SEATED FULL BODY STRETCHES

Seated full body stretches are a convenient and effective way for seniors to improve flexibility, reduce muscle tension, and enhance mobility while seated in a chair. These stretches can help increase blood flow, improve posture, and alleviate stiffness, making them an ideal option for those who may have mobility limitations or prefer a seated workout. Here are some seated Stretch:

- Sit tall in a chair with your shoulders relaxed.

- Gently tilt your head to one side, bringing your ear towards your shoulder, feeling a stretch in the side of your neck.

- Hold the stretch for 15-30 seconds, then switch sides and repeat.

2. Shoulder Roll:

- Sit tall with your arms relaxed at your sides.

- Roll your shoulders backward in a circular motion, lifting them up towards your ears, back, and down.

- Repeat the shoulder rolls for 10-15 repetitions, then reverse the direction.

3. Seated Cat-Cow Stretch:

- Sit on the edge of your chair with your hands on your knees.

- Inhale and arch your back, lifting your chest and gazing up (Cow Pose).

- Exhale and round your back, tucking your chin towards your chest (Cat Pose).

- Repeat the cat-cow stretch for 10-15 cycles to mobilize the spine.

4. Seated Side Stretch:

- Sit tall with your feet flat on the floor.

- Reach one arm overhead and lean towards the opposite side, feeling a stretch along the side of the body.

- Hold the stretch for 15-30 seconds, then switch sides and repeat.

5. Seated Forward Bend:

- Sit on the edge of your chair with your feet hip-width apart.

- Hinge at the hips and fold forward, reaching towards your toes or shins, feeling a stretch in the back of the legs (hamstrings).

- Hold the stretch for 15-30 seconds, then slowly sit back up.

6. Seated Spinal Twist:

- Sit tall with your feet planted on the floor and your hands on your thighs.

- Twist your torso to one side, placing one hand behind you and the other hand on the opposite thigh, feeling a gentle stretch in the spine and obliques.

- Hold the stretch for 15-30 seconds, then twist to the other side and repeat.

7. Seated Leg Extension Stretch:

- Sit tall with one leg extended out in front of you and the other knee bent.

- Reach towards your toes or ankle, feeling a stretch in the back of the extended leg (hamstrings).

- Hold the stretch for 15-30 seconds, then switch legs and repeat.

8. Seated Ankle Circles:

- Sit tall with your feet flat on the floor.

- Lift one foot off the ground and make circular motions with your ankle in a clockwise direction.

- Reverse the direction and make circles in a counterclockwise motion.

- Continue for 30 seconds, then switch feet and repeat.

Remember to move slowly and gently through each stretch, breathing deeply and focusing on relaxation. Hold each stretch for 15-30 seconds and repeat on both sides to target all major muscle groups in the body. Incorporate these seated full body stretches into your daily routine to improve flexibility, reduce muscle tension, and enhance overall mobility and function as a senior. Consult with a healthcare provider or fitness professional before starting any new exercise routine, especially if you have any underlying health conditions or concerns. Enjoy the benefits of seated full body stretches and keep your entire body strong, flexible, and mobile through regular stretching exercises from the comfort of a chair.

Standing Full Body Stretches for Seniors what

Standing full body stretches are a great way for seniors to improve flexibility, enhance circulation, and maintain range of motion throughout the body. These stretches can help alleviate muscle tension, improve balance, and promote better posture, making them an important component of a healthy and active lifestyle. Standing full body stretches can be easily incorporated into your daily routine and can be performed anywhere, making them a convenient option for seniors looking to improve their overall well-being. Here are some effective standing full body stretches for seniors to target all major muscle groups:

1. Arm Circles:

- Stand tall with your feet hip-width apart.

- Extend your arms out to the sides at shoulder height.

- Begin making small circles with your arms, gradually increasing the size of the circles.

- Reverse the direction of the circles after 10-15 repetitions.

2. Side Stretch:

- Stand with your feet hip-width apart and arms extended overhead.

- Lean to one side, feeling a stretch along the side of your body.

- Hold the stretch for 15-30 seconds, then switch sides and repeat.

3. Standing Quad Stretch:

- Stand tall with your feet hip-width apart.

- Bend one knee and bring your heel towards your glutes, grasping your ankle with your hand.

- Keep your knees close together and gently push your hip forward, feeling a stretch in the front of the thigh.

- Hold the stretch for 15-30 seconds, then switch legs and repeat.

4. Hamstring Stretch:

- Stand with your feet hip-width apart.

- Hinge at the hips and bend forward, reaching towards your toes or shins, feeling a stretch in the back of the legs (hamstrings).

- Hold the stretch for 15-30 seconds, then slowly come back up.

5. Chest Opener:

- Stand tall with your feet hip-width apart.

- Clasp your hands behind your back and straighten your arms, lifting them slightly and opening up the chest.

- Hold the stretch for 15-30 seconds, feeling a stretch in the chest and shoulders.

6. Standing Calf Stretch:

- Stand facing a wall with your hands resting on the wall for support.

- Step one foot back and press the heel into the floor, keeping the back leg straight.

- Lean forward into the stretch, feeling a stretch in the calf muscle of the back leg.

- Hold the stretch for 15-30 seconds, then switch legs and repeat.

7. Spinal Twist:

- Stand with your feet hip-width apart and arms extended out to the sides.

- Twist your torso to one side, bringing one arm across your body and the other arm behind you, feeling a stretch in the spine and obliques.

- Hold the stretch for 15-30 seconds, then twist to the other side and repeat.

8. Ankle Circles:

- Stand tall with your feet hip-width apart.

- Lift one foot off the ground and make circular motions with your ankle in a clockwise direction.

- Reverse the direction and make circles in a counterclockwise motion.

- Continue for 30 seconds, then switch feet and repeat.

Remember to breathe deeply and move mindfully through each stretch, focusing on proper alignment and avoiding any pain. Hold each stretch for 15-30 seconds and repeat on both sides to target all major muscle groups in the body. Incorporate these standing full body stretches into your daily routine to improve flexibility, reduce muscle tension, and enhance overall mobility and function as a senior. Consult with a healthcare provider or fitness professional before starting any new exercise routine, especially if you have any underlying health conditions or concerns. Enjoy the benefits of standing full body stretches and keep your entire body strong, flexible, and mobile through regular stretching exercises.

Chair-Assisted Full Body Stretches for Seniors

Chair-assisted full body stretches are a gentle and effective way for seniors to improve flexibility, reduce muscle tension, and enhance mobility while seated in a chair. These stretches can help increase blood flow, improve posture, and alleviate stiffness, making them an excellent option for those who may have limited mobility or balance issues. Chair-assisted stretches provide support and stability, making them safe and accessible for seniors of all fitness levels. Here are some chair-assisted full body stretches for seniors to target all major muscle groups:

1. Seated Shoulder Stretch:

- Sit tall in a chair with your feet flat on the floor.

- Bring one arm across your body and use the opposite hand to gently press the arm towards you, feeling a stretch in the shoulder and upper back.

- Hold the stretch for 15-30 seconds, then switch arms and repeat.

2. Seated Side Stretch:

- Sit tall with your feet planted on the floor.

- Reach one arm overhead and lean towards the opposite side, feeling a stretch along the side of the body.

- Hold the stretch for 15-30 seconds, then switch sides and repeat.

3. Seated Spinal Twist:

- Sit in a chair with your feet flat on the floor.

- Twist your torso to one side, placing one hand on the outside of the opposite thigh and the other hand on the back of the chair, feeling a stretch in the spine and obliques.

- Hold the stretch for 15-30 seconds, then twist to the other side and repeat.

4. Seated Hip Flexor Stretch:

- Sit on the edge of a chair with one foot flat on the floor and the other knee bent.

- Lean forward, keeping your back straight, and press into the bent knee, feeling a stretch in the front of the hip.

- Hold the stretch for 15-30 seconds, then switch legs and repeat.

5. Seated Hamstring Stretch:

- Sit tall with one leg extended in front of you and the other foot flat on the floor.

- Lean forward from the hips, reaching towards the extended leg, feeling a stretch in the back of the thigh (hamstrings).

- Hold the stretch for 15-30 seconds, then switch legs and repeat.

6. Seated Figure-four Stretch:

- Sit tall with your feet flat on the floor.

- Cross one ankle over the opposite knee and gently press down on the crossed knee, feeling a stretch in the hip and glutes.

- Hold the stretch for 15-30 seconds, then switch legs and repeat.

7. Seated Calf Stretch:

- Sit tall with your feet flat on the floor.

- Extend one leg out in front of you and place the heel on the floor, flexing the foot.

- Lean forward slightly, feeling a stretch in the calf muscle of the extended leg.

- Hold the stretch for 15-30 seconds, then switch legs and repeat.

8. Seated Neck Stretch:

- Sit tall with your shoulders relaxed.

- Tilt your head to one side, bringing your ear towards your shoulder, feeling a stretch in the side of the neck.

- Hold the stretch for 15-30 seconds, then switch sides and repeat.

Remember to breathe deeply and relax into each stretch, focusing on proper alignment and avoiding any pain. Hold each stretch for 15-30 seconds and repeat on both sides to target all major muscle groups in the body. Incorporate these chair-assisted full body stretches into your daily routine to improve flexibility, reduce muscle tension, and enhance overall mobility and function as a senior. Consult with a healthcare provider or fitness professional before starting any new exercise routine, especially if you have any underlying health conditions or concerns. Enjoy the benefits of chair-assisted full body stretches and keep your entire body strong, flexible, and mobile through regular stretching exercises from the comfort   of   a   chair.

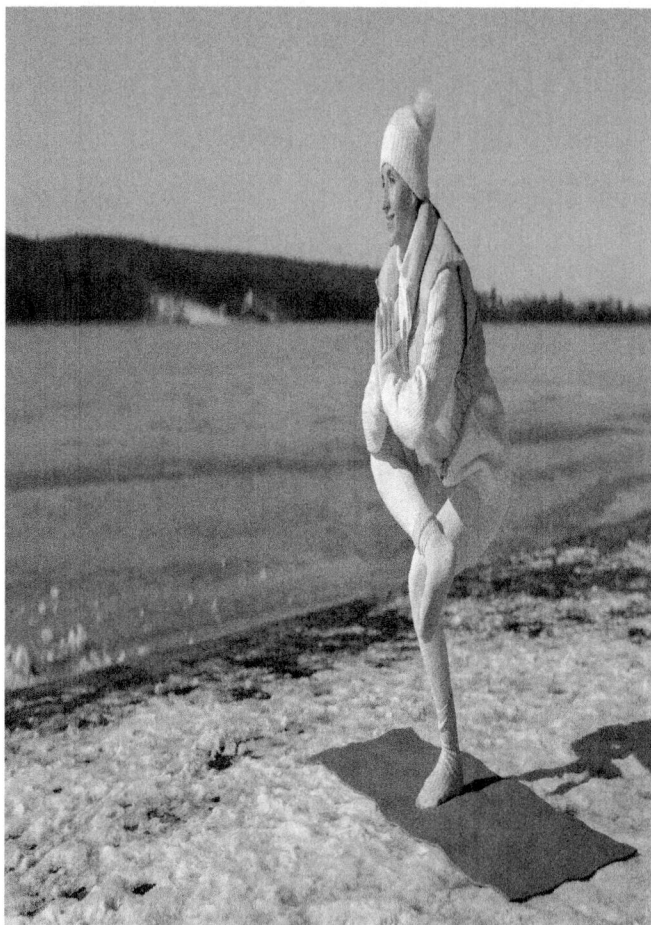

SIX:

ADDITIONAL TIPS FOR SENIORS

In addition to incorporating seated, standing, and chair-assisted full body stretches into your daily routine, there are several other tips and strategies that seniors can follow to improve their overall health and well-being:

1. Stay Active: Regular physical activity is essential for maintaining mobility, muscle strength, and cardiovascular health. In addition to stretching exercises, incorporate activities like walking, swimming, or gentle yoga to stay active and fit.

2. Practice Balance Exercises: Balance exercises can help prevent falls and improve stability. Simple exercises like standing on one leg or taking a tai chi class can help seniors improve their balance and coordination.

3. Maintain a Healthy Diet: Eating a balanced and nutritious diet is important for overall health and well-being. Seniors should focus on consuming a variety of fruits, vegetables, whole grains, lean proteins, and healthy fats to support their energy levels and immune function.

4. Stay Hydrated: Dehydration can contribute to a variety of health concerns, including fatigue, dizziness, and urinary tract infections. Seniors should aim to drink plenty of water throughout the day to stay hydrated and support their overall health.

5. Get Plenty of Sleep: Quality sleep is essential for physical and mental health. Seniors should aim to get 7-9 hours of sleep each night to support their immune function, cognitive abilities, and overall well-being.

6. Practice Mindfulness and Stress Management: Stress can have a negative impact on health and well-being. Seniors can benefit from practices like deep breathing, meditation, or gentle yoga to help reduce stress and promote relaxation.

7. Stay Socially Connected: Maintaining social connections is important for mental and emotional well-being. Seniors should make an effort to stay in touch with friends and family members, participate in community activities, or join clubs and organizations to stay socially engaged.

8. Visit Your Healthcare Provider Regularly: Regular check-ups with your healthcare provider are important for monitoring your health and addressing any concerns or issues that may arise. Seniors should schedule annual physicals, screenings, and vaccinations as recommended by their healthcare provider.

9. Stay Mentally Active: Keeping the mind sharp and engaged is important for cognitive function. Seniors can challenge their brains by reading, doing puzzles, learning new skills, or participating in educational activities to support mental acuity.

10. Listen to Your Body: Pay attention to your body's signals and adjust your activities and routines accordingly. If you experience pain, discomfort, or unusual symptoms, seek guidance from a healthcare provider or medical professional.

By incorporating these tips into your daily routine, seniors can enhance their overall health, well-being, and quality of life. Staying active, practicing healthy habits, and prioritizing self-care are essential components of successful aging. Remember to consult with your healthcare provider before starting any new exercise program or making significant changes to your lifestyle to ensure your safety and well-being.

Breathing Techniques for Stretching

Breathing plays a crucial role in enhancing the effectiveness of stretching exercises. Proper breathing techniques can help to relax the body, increase oxygen flow to the muscles, improve flexibility, and promote a greater sense of mindfulness during stretching routines. Here are some breathing techniques to incorporate into your stretching practice:

1. Deep Breathing: Deep breathing involves taking slow, deep breaths in through the nose, filling the lungs with air, and exhaling slowly through the mouth. Deep breathing helps to oxygenate the muscles, relax the mind and body, and reduce stress and tension. Practice deep breathing before, during, and after stretching exercises to help optimize your performance and maximize the benefits of your stretching routine.

2. Coordinated Breathing: Coordinating your breath with your movements can help to synchronize your body and mind during stretching exercises. Inhale as you lengthen or reach for a stretch, and exhale as you release or relax into the stretch. This rhythmic breathing pattern can enhance your focus, improve your range of motion, and facilitate deeper and more effective stretches.

3. Diaphragmatic Breathing: Diaphragmatic breathing, also known as belly breathing, involves breathing deeply into the diaphragm rather than shallow breathing into the chest. To practice diaphragmatic breathing, place one hand on your abdomen and the other hand on your chest. Inhale deeply through the nose, allowing the belly to rise as you fill the lungs with air, then exhale slowly through the mouth, drawing the belly in towards the spine. Diaphragmatic breathing can help to relax the body, reduce tension in the muscles, and support a more effective stretching experience.

4. Breath Holds: Incorporating breath holds into your stretching routine can help to deepen stretches, improve flexibility, and release tension in the muscles. To practice breath holds, take a deep breath in before moving into a stretch, hold your breath as you slowly stretch deeper into the pose, then exhale as you release and relax into the stretch. Hold the stretch for a few seconds before repeating the process on the other side. Breath holds can intensify the stretch and promote a greater sense of relaxation and release in the muscles.

5. Counting Breaths: Counting your breaths during stretching exercises can help to regulate your breathing, maintain focus, and control the pace of your movements. Inhale for a count of three or four as you prepare for a stretch, hold the breath for a count of one or two as you move deeper into the stretch, and exhale for a count of three or four as you release and relax into the pose. Counting your breaths can help to create a sense of rhythm and awareness in your stretching practice, enhancing the mind-body connection and optimizing the benefits of your stretching routine.

Incorporate these breathing techniques into your stretching practice to enhance the effectiveness of your stretches, promote relaxation, and support a deeper connection between your body and mind. Remember to listen to your body, breathe deeply and mindfully, and practice these breathing techniques with intention and awareness to maximize the benefits of your stretching routine. Consult with a healthcare provider or fitness professional before starting any new exercise program, especially if you have any underlying health conditions or concerns. Enjoy the benefits of incorporating proper breathing techniques into your stretching routine and experience the positive impact on your flexibility, mobility, and overall well-being.

How to Modify Stretches for Individual Needs

Stretching is a key component of a well-rounded fitness routine, but it's important to remember that not all stretches are suitable for everyone. Depending on factors such as age, fitness level, flexibility, and any existing injuries or conditions, modifications may be necessary to ensure safety and effectiveness. Here are some tips on how to modify stretches to meet individual needs:

1. Start Slow and Gradual: If you're new to stretching or have limited flexibility, it's important to start slow and gradual. Begin with gentle stretches and gradually increase the intensity and duration as your body becomes more accustomed to the movements. Listen to your body and avoid pushing yourself too hard too soon.

2. Focus on Proper Alignment: Proper alignment is crucial for safe and effective stretching. Pay attention to your posture, body positioning, and form during each stretch. Make sure to keep your spine neutral, engage your core muscles, and avoid unnecessary strain on your joints. If needed, use props like blocks, straps, or chairs to support your body and help maintain proper alignment.

3. Adjust Range of Motion: If a stretch feels too intense or uncomfortable, don't force yourself into a deep range of motion. Instead, adjust the position or movement to a level that feels challenging but manageable. For example, you can decrease the angle of a stretch, reduce the distance you reach, or modify the position of your limbs to make the stretch more accessible.

4. Modify for Injury or Condition: If you have a pre-existing injury or condition that limits your range of motion or mobility, it's essential to modify stretches accordingly. Consult with a healthcare provider or physical therapist to determine safe and appropriate modifications for your specific needs. They can provide guidance on which stretches to avoid, how to adapt movements to prevent further injury, and alternative exercises to support your recovery.

5. Use Props and Support: Props and support tools can be beneficial for modifying stretches and providing assistance for those with limited flexibility or mobility. Yoga blocks, straps, resistance bands, chairs, and bolsters can help you customize stretches to your individual needs, maintain proper alignment, and deepen the stretch without straining your muscles or joints.

6. Incorporate Gentle Movement: Instead of holding static stretches for an extended period, consider incorporating dynamic or flowing movements into your stretching routine. Gentle movements like circles, rotations, or pulsing can help improve flexibility, increase circulation, and reduce muscle tension while minimizing the risk of overstretching.

7. Listen to Your Body: Ultimately, the most important factor in modifying stretches for individual needs is listening to your body. Pay attention to how you feel during each stretch, identify areas of tension or discomfort, and adjust the intensity or position accordingly. Trust your instincts and make modifications that feel right for your body and overall well-being.

By applying these tips and techniques, you can tailor your stretching routine to meet your individual needs, improve flexibility, and prevent injury. Remember that everyone's body is unique, and it's important to honor your body's limitations and capabilities. Consult with a fitness professional or healthcare provider if you have any concerns or questions about modifying stretches to suit your individual needs. Enjoy the benefits of a personalized and safe stretching practice that supports your overall health and wellness goals.

Common Mistakes to Avoid in Stretching Exercises

Stretching is an important component of any fitness routine, helping to improve flexibility, prevent injury, and enhance performance. However, there are common mistakes that people often make during stretching exercises that can compromise their effectiveness and increase the risk of injury. Here are some common mistakes to avoid in stretching exercises:

1. Skipping Warm-up: One of the most common mistakes people make is skipping the warm-up before stretching. A proper warm-up helps to increase blood flow to the muscles, raise body temperature, and prepare the body for the stretching exercises. Without a warm-up, the muscles may be tight and less pliable, increasing the risk of strain or injury during stretching.

2. Bouncing or Jerking Movements: Bouncing or jerking movements during stretching, also known as ballistic stretching, can cause the muscles to tighten and potentially lead to injury. It's important to perform slow, controlled movements during stretches to allow the muscles to gradually lengthen and relax.

3. Holding Your Breath: Holding your breath while stretching can increase tension in the body and limit the effectiveness of the stretch. Proper breathing techniques, such as deep breathing and coordinated breath with movements, can help to relax the body, improve oxygen flow to the muscles, and enhance the benefits of stretching.

4. Overstretching: It's important to stretch to the point of tension, not pain. Overstretching can cause muscle strains, ligament damage, and joint instability. Listen to your body and respect your limits when stretching, gradually increasing the intensity and duration of the stretch over time.

5. Ignoring Muscle Imbalances: Muscle imbalances, where certain muscles are tight and others are weak, can affect your overall flexibility and posture. It's important to address muscle imbalances through targeted stretching and strengthening exercises to improve flexibility and prevent injury.

6. Holding Static Stretches Too Long: Holding static stretches for excessively long periods, especially without proper warm-up or cooldown, can lead to muscle fatigue and decrease muscle performance. Aim to hold each stretch for 15-30 seconds and repeat multiple times, gradually increasing the stretch intensity as your muscles loosen up.

7. Neglecting Major Muscle Groups: It's common for people to focus on stretching certain areas of the body, such as the hamstrings or quadriceps, while neglecting other major muscle groups. A well-rounded stretching routine should target all major muscle groups, including the back, shoulders, hip flexors, and calves, to maintain overall flexibility and prevent imbalances.

8. Rushing Through Stretches: Rushing through stretches without proper form or attention to detail can reduce the effectiveness of the stretch and increase the risk of injury. Take your time with each stretch, focus on proper alignment and technique, and concentrate on relaxing and releasing tension in the muscles.

9. Not Tailoring Stretches to Individual Needs: Everyone's body is different, and stretching routines should be tailored to individual needs, including age, fitness level, flexibility, and any existing injuries or conditions. Avoid following a one-size-fits-all approach to stretching and instead customize your stretches to suit your body and goals.

10. Failing to Listen to Your Body: The most important mistake to avoid in stretching exercises is failing to listen to your body. Pay attention to how your body feels during each stretch, respect your limits, and modify or stop any stretches that cause pain or discomfort. Communicate with a fitness professional or healthcare provider if you have any concerns or questions about your stretching routine.

By avoiding these common mistakes and practicing safe and effective stretching techniques, you can improve flexibility, reduce the risk of injury, and enhance the benefits of your stretching routine. Remember to prioritize proper warm-up, breath control, controlled movements, and individualized stretches to optimize your stretching exercises and support your overall fitness goals. Consult with a fitness professional or healthcare provider if you have any questions or need guidance on safe and effective stretching practices.

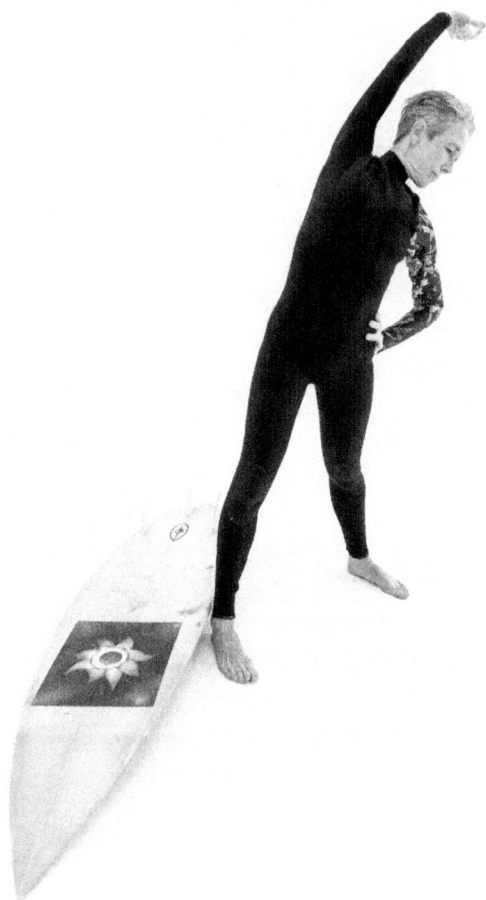

Conclusion

In conclusion, stretching is a valuable and beneficial practice for seniors that can have a significant impact on their overall health and well-being. By incorporating stretching exercises into their daily routine, seniors can experience a wide range of benefits that contribute to improved flexibility, mobility, and quality of life.

Recap of the Benefits of Stretching for Seniors:

1. Improved Flexibility: Regular stretching helps to maintain and increase flexibility in muscles, joints, and connective tissues, which can enhance range of motion and reduce the risk of injury.

2. Enhanced Mobility: Stretching exercises can improve balance, coordination, and posture, making everyday movements easier and more comfortable for seniors.

3. Reduced Muscle Tension: Stretching helps to alleviate muscle tightness and tension, promoting relaxation, stress relief, and improved muscle function.

4. Injury Prevention: Stretching can help prevent injuries by increasing muscle elasticity, improving joint stability, and supporting proper alignment and posture.

5. Improved Circulation: Stretching exercises promote better blood flow to the muscles and tissues, which can enhance circulation, boost energy levels, and support overall cardiovascular health.

Encouragement to Incorporate Stretching into Daily Routine:

I strongly encourage seniors to incorporate stretching into their daily routine as a simple and effective way to promote physical and mental well-being. Whether done in the morning to wake up the body, throughout the day to relieve tension and stiffness, or in the evening to relax and unwind, stretching can be a valuable and enjoyable practice for seniors of all ages and fitness levels. Remember to start slowly, listen to your body, and modify stretches to suit your individual needs and abilities.

committing to a regular stretching routine, seniors can experience the numerous benefits of improved flexibility, mobility, and overall health. Whether done independently or as part of a structured exercise program, stretching can be a powerful tool for enhancing quality of life, promoting independence, and supporting healthy aging. So, why not take the first step today and incorporate stretching into your daily routine? Your body will be grateful for it. Stretch, breathe, and move with intention, and enjoy the positive impact that stretching can have on your body, mind, and spirit.

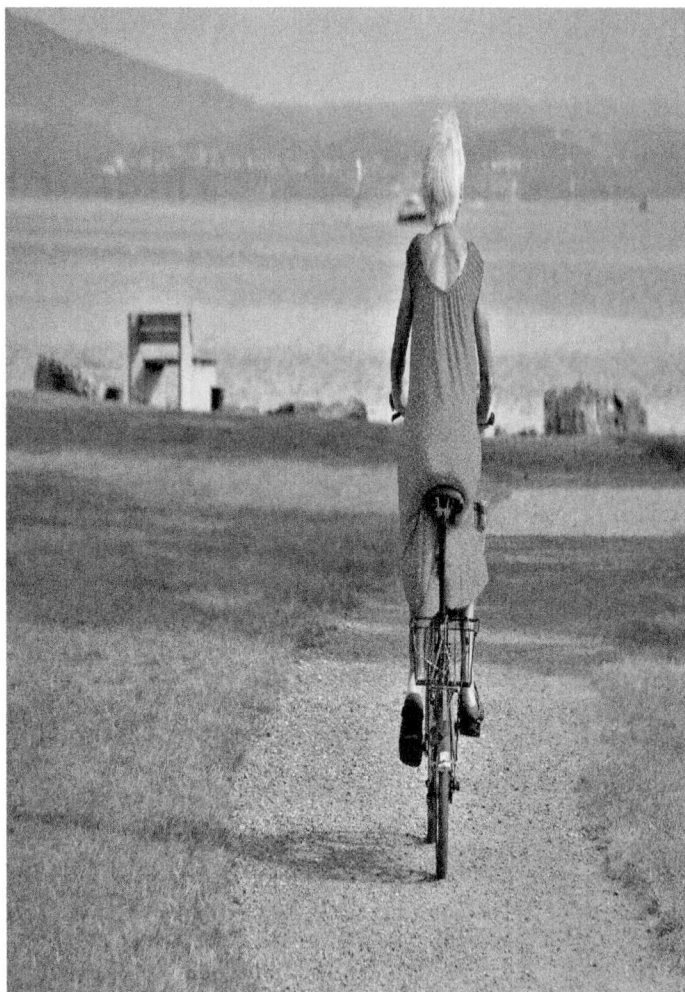

Printed in Dunstable, United Kingdom